Table of Contents

For all my sista souljahs
who wear their naps proudly

IN THE BEGINNING

When your illusions are shattered, you grow up. The time has come for illusions and delusions about the natural hair mystique to be looked at with a cold eye and the truth to be told. First, I should say that I am natural. But I also believe in telling the truth to help with our hair and the truth is that far too many naturals are in hair crisis and deep denial.

In America, where black on black crime is holocaustic, lack of education, miseducation, homelessness, and lack of jobs abound; what is the biggest issue among black women? HAIR!! In this author's opinion the so called natural hair movement is the worst and most divisive thing to happen to Black America since the Willie Lynch letter. It is the worst bamboozling of black people since the forty acres and a mule lie.

Being followers, as many are, black women have been led down a path that they knew nothing about and many grew to hate. So, they returned to the comfort of relaxing their hair. To the comfort of two or three products and no schisms. If they knew the truth and how to take care of their natural hair, this would not and will not happen. Many women have always been natural, but gaining curls was never their quest. This book in no way reflects all naturals. Just far too many from what I have observed.

Daily, there are debates and fights online about hair that surely, if these ladies were in each other's presence, there would be literal scuffles on the floor. There are sects and subgroups that separate the "wavy or curly" from the "nappy" and definitions upon definitions of what a "true" natural is. As well as ostracizing from one group to the next according to what angers them. What started this madness?

When the documentary "Good Hair" was released, many black women decided that relaxers were literally killing them and decided to go natural with their hair. I found it utterly fascinating that a comedian, not anyone in the hair field at all, could actually shape the mentality of American black women about our hair. I was not surprised however, because we are a nation of followers. From rappers and musicians to entertainers, we follow the prevailing wind. In the absence of our ability to think and lead ourselves, they set the tone in so many areas of our lives. From ass-dragging pants to our vernacular to names of our kids, you name it, we do it. Well, some do. Some, like myself, are not followers. Good, bad, or indifferent, we think for ourselves.

My going natural is not a political choice or because of the urging of anyone else. I went natural because I became known to a degree, on social media, as a hair growth specialist and my inbox begin to fill up with questions, concerns, and complaints about natural hair. When the time came for me to relax my new growth, I cut it instead. I wanted to know what was causing so many issues for my natural hair sisters. This was the only way that I could see and decide if I could offer help.

I am going to get the "relaxer scare" out of the way and then focus on the main. Now, the truth is that damage occurs in relaxers when they are done incessantly, not allowing enough time between relaxer treatments. Damage also occurs when women decide to do apply their own relaxers instead of going to a professional. They apply relaxers that are often too strong for their hair or they leave it in too long, thinking, "if I let it stay on longer it will get really straight" or they relax the whole head of hair over each time they need their roots retouched. These things lead to over-processing and weak hair that will break. Bleaching also is a hair killer, especially when you are relaxed. All of the above will continually be practiced, but many will never admit guilt in any of the above.

This is what happens if the truth were told, but many naturals are not at all fond of the truth about hair and are often in denial. A denial that they will fight vehemently over. There are lies upon lies told every day about their hair, not realizing that help can only come with the truth.

Relaxers are not the "boogeyman". The ingredient that frightens women is sodium hydroxide also known as lye. However, it is safe when handled and applied properly. The neutralizing shampoo also lowers the pH balance of the hair and reforms the cystine bonds. Women who relax their hair knew about this ingredient all along, but the documentary made it appear as though a vat of pure lye was taken from the factory and dumped on their heads. We see and hear, but we don't really listen.

The great fear of fibroid tumors is another concern and some tests prove that fibroids are usually genetic. There is no proof that relaxers cause them, because we then have to wonder why white women and women in general had them long before such a thing as relaxers were invented.

But lye is one of the ingredients. I always tell my relaxed and natural clients to check the ingredient list when buying hair products, or anything for that matter. If the main ingredients that you are buying the product for is not listed in the third or fourth position, then it is masked in a lot of other ingredients.

For those who think that sodium hydroxide is just dumped on the head as it chews their hair and scalp away, it is not the most prominent ingredient in relaxers. Not to mention that is applied to the hair and not the scalp. The neutralizing process stops the action of the relaxers and reforms the chemical bonds that are broken down during the process. You then go into a good hair care regimen to get and keep it healthy. Sodium hydroxide is not Pac Man, it does not continue to munch away at the hair as some seem to think. While it is a strong chemical, as many are that we use daily, the main thing to understand is that proper handling and replenishing the hair after it has been done is needed by some ladies to control an otherwise unattractive mane.

Sodium hydroxide is also used quite a bit in food processing. The compound is often used in steps for peeling fruits and vegetables, processing cocoa and chocolate, thickening of ice cream, poultry scalding and soda processing. Olives are soaked in sodium hydroxide along with other substances to make them black, and soft pretzels are also coated with the compound to give them a chewy texture. It is also an ingredient in refined coconut oil and body soaps. People have taken a little information from a documentary and run with it. Never considering deeper research, like how it is ingested into our bodies. Don't use it to relax your hair, but eating it is fine. Thoroughly ironic.

While there is absolutely nothing wrong with wearing your hair natural. It can be a beautiful thing. You need your heart in it, time, care and above all, patience. Relaxed hair can be beautiful and healthy, also. Thanks can be given to the natural craze because it brought forth many products to help to keep relaxed hair even healthier.

Hair is ornamental and is made to be beautiful on your head in the fashion you choose. Altering the hair is no different than altering anything else about your looks that you were born with and felt you wanted to alter or improve on. If you were born with warts and at some time you decided to get them removed to make yourself look better, who is to say you are wrong? Not that anyone would. But when it comes to hair, black women in America are obsessed and divisive to the point of it being a topic vehemently discussed daily with battles to rival the Civil War.   With the state of the black community being what it is in America, this is a tragedy. It is hair, not world peace. I have a problem when people are supposed to be promoting self-love and spewing venom towards others. In my opinion, this behavior is steeped in self-hate.

CRASH OF THE NATURAL MYSTIQUE

At this point, I can already feel the flames flickering about my ears. Why? Because from what I have witnessed for five years, the truth is the last thing many naturals want to hear. They want the myths and miracles. Both are destructive to our hair. I am the truth, as they say, "the real MVP" that will not appease us to our detriment. If I could grab and shake the hell out of the myth and miracle ladies and scream "wake up", I would. I should mention that many other naturals feel the same way.

In 2012, I decided to cut my long, healthy, relaxed hair for one reason: the incessant inquiries from natural hair wearers about their troubled hair and how to get and retain length. The inquiries were often inboxed to me through my Facebook account or email. I had written My Hair Won't Grow and gained a following of women who wanted to achieve what I had, which was waist length hair. My hair was relaxed at the time and these ladies knew it, so they stealthily wrote to me in a way that would not call attention to them. I had no problem helping them or any woman in this endeavor, including women from Africa and other countries. Indeed, it was my pleasure.

About two years into my quest to see if, being natural, I could achieve waist length hair and to see what was causing so much angst among naturals, I decided to join some natural hair groups on Facebook. I also wanted to learn from them about caring for naturals. No one knows it all about hair. I worked my way into the groups slowly by giving advice and tips on hair growth. I wanted to help, where before, I had no interest in natural hair or what they thought about my relaxed hair. I was proud of their pride and wanted to help and to learn even more about natural hair care.

Because I was natural I was welcomed, but I also still had my beauty shop and mostly did relaxed hair. I was somewhat forced to endure the assault on ladies who still relaxed their hair or wore it straight. Well, except for Oprah and Michelle O. You just didn't berate those ladies. The assaults puzzled me because the mantra of these ladies was, "I love my natural hair." If you love your hair or anything about yourself what was the incessant need to censure other ladies about their hair choices. They seemed to have perms/relaxers on the brain and this, too, was puzzling in a sort of "thou doth protest too loudly" way. They often posted pictures of women with scalp abnormalities like dissecting cellulitis and saying relaxers did it. Why? This is a scalp disease, dissecting cellulitis, has nothing to do with relaxers or any particular race. Why the need to post and blame relaxers for it? I have seen it posted many, many times as relaxer damage. This escapes me, truly.

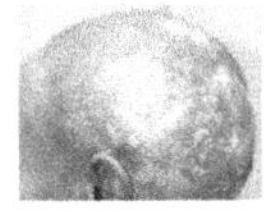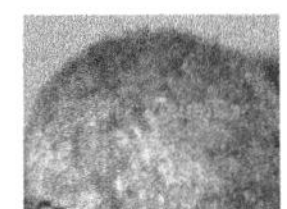

This was just one of the errors made. Many of them seemed bitter and angry with their onslaught of negativity toward anyone who did not make the same choice as they had, even as a natural. The fights, cussing among each other, was beyond absurd. I was so disappointed. I could not see the beauty of the natural hair because of the deluge of ugliness being spewed. As a people who were once enslaved and oppressed, the very idea of trying to take away even the most minute freedom or choice is deplorable. These people with their constant rants and memes put me off in such a way that words escape me. I coined a phrase for them many years ago, they are called Natural Nazis.

Though I have never been one to be into colorism, I could not help but notice that most, not all, of these women were unattractive, dark-complected, and had the kinkiest or nappiest hair on their heads. To me and others, it did not seem like love of self but reeked of self-hatred. I soon began to realize that secretly, many of them actually hated their hair. They were jealous of the ladies with long and/or curly hair. It was almost palpable. Now and then, just to see where people's heads were, I would post pictures of relaxed hair and say it was a natural blowout. Oh, the likes! Later, I would post a beautiful head of long, silky, relaxed hair and it would be virtually ignored. Why? Because they cannot admit the truth, must hold on to the lies. Healthy hair is healthy hair. Both natural and relaxed hair can be very beautiful and healthy. But that thing within will not allow some naturals to say it. Especially in front of other naturals. Hypocrisy!

When other women and I posted pictures of our long hair, it was met with mostly disbelief that it was actually our own root hair. Often we were accused of having weave. That in itself was an insult to all black women because it was saying that we are incapable of such growth. Some envied, but envy is a different mindset than jealousy. Mostly, it seemed they would rather have curly hair. Most natural hair pictures posted were altered curly hair.

I must point out that some of the ladies never did this. They were proud of their own hair, and it showed in their attitude. They absolutely agreed that because they chose natural, it did not mean that all women should. They were very much outnumbered, however.

There was always talk of hair crushes. A glaring indication of not being happy with their own. The hair crush at one time, when being natural was real, uniting, powerful, and awe-inspiring, was Angela Davis. I remember all of those beautiful afros and the absolute pride of wearing them. Our hair was nappy and we truly loved It. But now the hair crush has become a mixed race woman with curly hair, Tracee Ross. That in itself speaks volumes.

Over time, I began to realize what a Gordian knot the natural hair frenzy was comprised of. These women easily tear each other apart when one does not agree with the next. It is not a state of beauty but of perpetual feelings of being unattractive and hate of their dark skin (even not so dark) and their nappy hair.

So many now are offended by the term "nappy" and have taken on the term whites have always used to describe their coils, "kinky". Who is trying to be white with that one? Talk about appropriation! They heat up a post when whites take what we think belongs to us, but steal their term for tight coils. A friend of mine said that the only ones who hate the term nappy are the ones with nappy hair. From my observances, I have to agree with him.

There are hair groups where the word "nappy" is forbidden and you will be kicked out immediately for using it. I left before they kicked my nappy-headed, and prone to say such, self out of there. I love the term nappy. It is derived from the term nap, as in the soft nap of carpet, and it is another distinction for us. I find no insult in it at all. However, it has become yet another debate to direct us away from the important issues that we should be focusing on.

Are we in America or what? We are Americans, not Africans, as one of the Africans in a natural hair group pointed out by saying, "when you visit our country, we call you Americans." The "our" indicating that it is not our, Americans, country. But many missed that word and her meaning. We turn the faucet off when the knowledge does not suit our state of mind. In this author's opinion the turning off of the faucet has caused hair to stagnate and put millions of dollars into "product frenzy" that end up under the sink in bathrooms. I have seen pictures of girls who have more products in their homes than I do in my beauty shop. Do we really think that corporations are in board meetings thinking, "What can we do for hair health and growth of black people's hair in America?" Or are they thinking, "The thirst is gargantuan, let's get that money!" Or more intelligently, "The natural hair movement is something we can definitely capitalize on." And they absolutely have.

At the end of this book I will list some products and you can decide whether we are targets, whether it is too much. Especially since the same hair issues prevail. I feel safe in saying that they, too, visit YouTube and see the "grow hair fast" or "grow your hair an inch in one week" videos. These videos get millions of views because the desperation is real as is the disappointment because it is simply not true. But corporations see our desperation. The scam artists do, too. I have seen some get "taken" with fake pictures and videos. They send money and receive no product at all or hair grease with a dash of one of the essential oils. It is tragic. Someone can post a picture of long hair and say horse pee made my hair grow and the question then becomes, "Where you get it? Can you buy it?"

Genetics, mostly, determine how fast your hair will grow each month. The average black woman's hair grows between a fourth and a third of an inch per month and most will grow around four inches a year. Asian hair generally grows faster and retains more length, as do Native Americans because many have coarse, straight hair. If you retain that length, not tear the ends off, which is where length is lost, in two years you will have eight inches, three years, a foot, and so on. Some may grow one half inch per month, but it is extremely rare that it will grow an inch per month, extremely rare. This is a truth that causes hands to cover ears and brains to go into delete mode.

We simply cannot let go of the dream, the illusion or delusion as we continue our quest for the "holy grail" of hair growth. It simply does not exist. If it did, there would be no need for the ceaseless changing of products or the plethora of wasted products that get used once and discarded when the miracle does not occur. If there was such a product, everyone would have it.

We need to get one thing cemented in our brains and that is: HAIR GROWS. Unless you have a physical issue, your head yields new growth every month as seen when you color or when you relax. That is your growth, at the root. The problem is that it is torn off on the ends as fast as it comes in at the root. End hair is older and has endured more and is apt to break faster. Notice how many ladies' long hair comes to a point of thinness as it gets close to the ends, same with ponytails. That is because it is broken. Great care should be given to the ends as well as the scalp. There should be less manipulation and staying away from curling and flat irons.

Products are to enhance hair health as it grows, but it does not make your hair grow. Say this in hair groups and be ready for a fight or to get booted. This truth is monumental and monumentally rejected. They simply cannot handle it. It shatters all illusions. It means that now, they have to work with their nap/kinks and who went natural for that? So, what happens? Wigs and weaves and braids (edge killers) because the hair just won't comply with our wishes. The sale of weave and wigs have skyrocketed since the natural hair movement. I find that interesting.

THE BIG LIE

Your natural hair is generally healthier than relaxed hair. However, relaxed hair can be healthy and thriving. If you are a true natural and your natural hair is virgin it can be very healthy or it can be very damaged. Why the "craze" of natural hair wearers? If the truth was told, as I said before, we are a nation of followers, and many went natural because of that.

Going natural is great if you intend to put in the work to keep it vibrant and healthy. Natural hair requires a commitment. But what we see far too often is unkempt, dirty, and linty hair. Fifteen different lengths of hair on one head. But post a picture of these disasters and the comments are "beautiful." Come on now! The comments are made simply to keep them in the natural camp. They should be told the truth and still kept in the camp. All natural hair is not beautiful. Just like all relaxed hair is not beautiful. Beautiful hair is healthy hair and many fall far short of that.

When naturals are "recruiting" they make it sound like hair nirvana and anything else is the devil. It is like the old saying, "there is nothing worse than a reformed whore." They slapped relaxers in their hair in a flash, but now they don't. So now, they want to preach the virtues of not relaxing to everyone else. The truth is that most natural hair requires work. The nappier it is, the more work is required. Many went natural thinking that this was "it" only to find great disappointment and scampered back to relaxing.

One thing I must also say, I am in both natural and relaxed hair groups. In relaxed groups, it is much more calm and the ladies much happier with their relaxed hair. It shows that something is wrong with the "love" that rarely shows up among naturals in their groups. Naturals, well some, also like to think that relaxed girls envy their hair. That is not true, but they love to think it. I am not sure why.

Girls who love relaxed hair, love their relaxed hair, and give no thought to naturals one way or another, know none of the lingo, nothing, except knowing that it is something that they absolutely do not want. And that is their right, to do with their hair as they please without the negativity and venom being spewed at them by Natural Nazis. I mean, what is it to the next woman how that woman wears her hair? Basically, it is none of your business.

Another thing not told to ladies before they go natural is the hours and hours and products and products needed to make the hair look great. I remember the days of wash, plait, and pick. The pain of untangling and breakage that leaves them with torn up hair. I was sick one time and did not detangle my hair for five days. When I say, it hurt me to my soul, it did. But I still pressed on and remained natural because I love it and to help other naturals.

I do admire the ladies who are true naturals and feel no need to twist, rod, and search for ways to make their hair not look nappy.

They are indeed happy with the glory God gave them from birth. They truly celebrate their blackness.

I have seen many who did the "big chop" and proudly proclaimed it via social media, but that is the last time you see their natural hair. The next pictures are mostly weaves or wigs. Straight or soft curl weaves, by the way. Hypocrisy. You never see their natural hair again because they found out what seasoned naturals already know. Being natural is not easy, especially when you climb the hair type chart into the 4's. Or as some have admitted, they were ashamed to go in public with their naps.

Many go back to relaxed and will not openly admit it, but they inbox me. I could not even imagine caring that much about the opinion of others about MY hair. But I do admit that the assault can be brutal from naturals. I have noticed as time moved on in the "movement" that it is not as bad. Why? Because so many naturals are weaving, wigging, texturizing, and cannot truly claim or explain why they wear the straight hair that they say mirrors our wanting to be "white". Of course, I do not go for that.

Time and inventions call for improvements in all areas of life. If relaxing or texturizing your hair makes your life or lifestyle easier, then that is your right. Again, we are Americans. Free. This was an actual conversation that I had with a couple.

Me: "How do you like your lady's natural look?"

Man: "It's okay."

Lady: "He doesn't touch my hair since I went natural and I think he doesn't say anything because I like it."

Man: "Honestly, it's the grease, I can't stand it. I just don't wanna put my hands in all that grease. I don't want it on my face either."

Lady: "You will be alright."

And he will. I have seen this talk before in hair groups, but I wanted to talk to people and get their views about it.

Of course, there were pros and cons. Most women said that it made women look like dudes. Some men also said that they do not want their woman looking like a man. Personally, I love very short hair and until it grows out, there are options. Many loved the natural look, if not for themselves, on other women.

Our natural hair is much more beautiful when it is shampooed and well moisturized. Being natural for too many is an excuse to be lazy about their hair care. It is obvious when you see them and especially sad when it is a child. They don't shampoo or cleanse the hair for months at a time, if ever. This prompted a girl to say once, "If you don't clean your hair, you don't clean your ass. That's just nasty." This is one of the things many men and women hate about the natural look. Of course, many love it, regardless. As with all things American.

CURL CHASERS

Ahh, the curl chasers. If I have heard this once, I have heard it a thousand times. "How can I get curls in my natural hair?" According to what the "movement" is about, getting back to our African roots, our over four hundred years removed African roots. So, why do you want curly hair? Wavy hair? Hypocrisy! Something is so very wrong about that. We spend hours rodding, braiding, plaiting, and twisting our natural hair so that it does not look African. It seems that the very last thing some of us want is a head of nappy hair. So we chase curls. Faux, false, or fake curls. We want curly or wavy, but definitely not nappy. And we justify it to ourselves, comfort ourselves by saying, "that is just a style." No, you have altered the natural hair, your root hair, because it is unattractive to you in its natural state. Might as well have a Jheri Curl.

I have seen staunch advocates of natural hair don a straight hair weave or wig and instantly began to throw and turn quickly to make it move. It is like they morphed into another person, so very happy to throw that straight hair. Hypocrisy! Women love to change. Wearing weaves, wigs, etc. is fine, but when you change with the "styles" ...hmm, picture out of focus.

They have hundreds of videos on YouTube to help them in their quest to be un-natural. It may seem harsh to say these things, but like with family, they are my people, I can talk about it and it is time someone spoke the truth. It isn't wearing a curly style. There is nothing wrong with that. It is thinking you can only be seen with a curly look. It is never wearing your root hair (meaning all yours from the root) unaltered. If you won't do this, you are perpetrating a lie. Total hypocrisy.

I have also seen many naturals who flat iron their hair. Again, nothing is wrong with that. But they holler about relaxed girls "wanting to look white." There are tons of videos where they are swinging and swaying their hair so hard and loving that "white girl" look, that you think they are going to get whiplash. Then there are the many before and after pictures of girls with their true natural hair looking sullen and smiling like they're in a toothpaste commercial once flat ironed. Hypocrisy!

They like to scare people with claims of "heat damage" from flat irons, but what they won't tell is the truth. Women get their hair flat ironed and hit the humidity, and it puffs. So the next day they flat iron it again and the day after and the day after, and you simply can't do that. That is where heat damage comes in. My suggestion is a scarf or hat until you get inside, go straight to the restroom and come out fabulous. When the day or event is over, wrap it back up!

There is nothing wrong with flat ironing, but if you do, they put you in the "not so natural" camp. How can you with your hair rodded to death, plaited to death, twisted to death, call a sister out for flat ironing? Hypocrisy!

One of the most curious and unbelievable things I witnessed in natural hair groups was when a young natural lady that many followed and bought her book, decided that taking care of her natural hair was too great a chore for her, and she relaxed her hair. You would have thought Michelle Obama had died. It was her hair! Her choice! What did it take away from me or them? Nothing! If there was any lesson there it was stop being followers. As I said before, many have done the same. They went back to what worked best for them. Some have gone back to relaxing and decided natural was really what they wanted and did the "big chop" again. There are some who also let their natural hair get length only to have enough length to relax it again.

If I have seen this once, I have seen it a thousand times. Girls saying, "I HAD to big chop again." Why? Because their supposed healthy hair had become so damaged. I am sure, going in, this was not what they expected. Many have been honest and said this. Again, these are all taken from real life discussions among naturals.

PROTECTIVE STYLES?

Yes, the hair needs a rest from manipulation at times. Some women need protection from themselves. They do not have the knowledge or will not receive knowledge that will help to keep from breaking the hair. There are some styles that I consider as protective, like braids, if the edges are not strained and human hair is used. Synthetic hair changes the texture of your natural hair and braiding can cause you to retain length because the hair is growing undisturbed by brushing, combing, ironing, etc. But braids can also thin the hair.

The truth is most of these "styles" are weaves or wigs. Why? Because we still want the waist length, butt length, long, straight, wavy hair because we are repelled by the naps we see in the mirror. So we gave it a name. Protective. Hypocrisy!

Sew-in weaves can be destructive to your hair and edges, causing permanent traction alopecia, balding, and thinning when worn too much. A break is always needed when you weave, at least two weeks. You should also do a deep conditioner before and after. But saying that you are wearing a weave because you are protecting your hair is a fallacy, especially if it is not in professional, caring hands.

Again, your hair grows anyway, and a zillion products are unnecessary. When I posted my four year growth, the first thing always asked was, "What product did you use?" I absolutely cringed. I tell them that I am not much into products. For me, less

is more than enough.

TO BE OR NOT TO BE..who is natural?

There is not a week that goes by that this battle is not waged. If you color your hair, you are not natural. I beg to differ because color or not, the naps are still there. It may be a different color, but just as hard to deal with, just as hard to untangle and you dare not go to bed on that colored nappy hair unless you want to pay for it in the morning. The truth is none of our hair is chemical free. Unless you make and grow your own products, there are chemicals in them. But the girl who colors surely cannot put down the girl who perms. Then there are the "naturals" who relax just their edges. Whose child are they? Yes, coloring, relaxing, relaxing edges are all chemical processes.

Bleaching, in my opinion, is the most damaging thing you can do to your hair. Yet, I see so many blonde naturals. Kind of an oxymoron. Hypocrisy! Another divisive issue. Why? Does it really matter as long as the person is happy with their hair? It is hair, something ornamental to be played with and made beautiful as it suits the wearer.

As much as naturals accuse relaxed girls of wanting to look "white", which can never be, their constant altering of their true natural hair to waves and curls reeks of something definitely not quite black.

I also find it amazing that we are trying to go "African" when they buy as much weave as Americans. Seems many of them don't want to be nappy either. I have had African ladies to tell me that their husbands do not like natural hair and they relax theirs.

I love my natural hair. It can be totally gorgeous. But far too many with natural hair are looking like they did before we discovered hair care products. There is no excuse for that. We all have heard the "Miss Celie" remarks, but sometimes naturals bring the insults on themselves. A teen told me that she just got tired of a girl slamming her relaxed hair and one day told her, "Hey, I'm good. See this?", as she whipped her hair across her face, "I would rather have this than that ball of ground up hamburger meat you got on your head." Things like this are so unnecessary. We should leave each person to their choice.

THE DARKER THE BERRY?

This has little to do with natural hair, but I feel it bears mentioning as our skin color and hair often intertwine. The axiom continues "the sweeter the juice," not, "the more beautiful." I am not sure who has sickened our state of mind to believe that dark black is not beautiful black, but some think this and it shows, whether spoken or not. I have a hair group that I post hairstyle selfies, mine and other artist's work, in. I want to be fair because our rainbow has many hues. Our hair has many types and there is immense beauty among our people. I realized while searching for hairstyles that most of the ladies were fair or brown skinned as many are and have been in and on the covers of black magazines. Even the darker celebrities' skin color had been altered to the point of almost being unrecognizable. I never understood this. Maybe it is because my family had the rainbow. So, color of skin was not discussed. I never discussed it with my children, either.   One of my dear Facebook friends said, "It is because we are the middle child. They don't count us."

As far as I am concerned, we are all in this thing together. Deluding yourself otherwise is foolish and can be dangerous. If you don't believe it, get caught in the wrong place at the wrong time, in Alabama. You are then no longer light or dark, but the N word.

However, Facebook and Google helped me in my search to find dark beauties. I went to the pages that featured only dark girls and found some stunningly beautiful black women. In my opinion, there is no one more beautiful than a dark skinned beauty. Their beauty is enviable. But when I posted some of them, I began to notice that there were much fewer likes or comments. No matter our skin color, the hair can be from type 1 to type 4. Even when the picture was of a dark beauty with wavy natural hair, she still fell short on likes or comments. If she had a simple afro, she was basically ignored.

When I post these pictures, I never point out her dark skin, because that is obvious and I know that many dark skinned girls absolutely hate that lopsided compliment. "You are a pretty black girl," or "You are pretty to be dark skinned." Beauty is beauty! It does not need to be qualified, especially in an insulting manner clothed in a compliment. Simply saying, "You are a beautiful woman," will suffice.

Lighter does not mean more beautiful, as seen by too many unattractive (putting it mildly) white people. I do not know where the idea that lighter is better and beautiful came from, but I would throw it on the heap of trash that burns high among the many totally self-defacing ideas that black America has kept for centuries. Even Willie Lynch did not say light was better, though he helped to formulate it in the minds of our people. But good God! Willie Lynch has been dead for centuries.

Why then do we still perpetuate this ignorance? There is no excuse for it. We truly are our own worst enemies. We like nothing better than to verbally destroy, especially successful black women, like Beyonce. She is a favorite whipping girl of black women. They act like she owes them money or something. I am not a fan of her music, but have participated favorably in some of these assaults. Jealous much? I think so. If we can't rise above something that is centuries old and should be as dead as Willie Lynch is, will we ever be a thriving, united people? Do we even want to? I wonder.

PAY ATTENTION!

In spite of my chiding, I am a professional whose hair has reached waist length, relaxed and natural. So, in spite of the stubbornness and denial, I still help when I can. We are being targeted in ads, commercials, and infomercials. We need to pay attention. Look carefully at the hair that they are trying to say you, too, can have. If the camera pans away and comes back to straight hair, no. If the hair is already blown out before flat straightening, no. Will the product take you from post-shampoo (dried after conditioner and no blowing) to what you see on the screen? Probably not, unless your hair is in the 1, 2 or 3 group, and sometimes not 3.

Most of the women in those ads, like most of the YouTube ladies, have curly hair. But somehow we incessantly watch them, do as they do, expecting the same result, only to be disappointed. Be realistic! Care for your hair according to your type. Never look at ads of white girls or curly black girls and think it will work for your 4c hair. That is the hype to sell and make you hope for something totally unrealistic.

As for the ads and such, they pay marketers to know how to target you. They are very aware of the thirst. Pay attention! Don't just look and jump for the product, grabbing your phone or PC and ordering pronto. Watch it several times because you may miss it at first. When ladies post extraordinary, super-fast growth, you don't have to pay attention. It is simply not true. People lie on the net everyday about their hair. Lies about why it came out, what grew it out and how fast. It takes time, care and patience to achieve growth. There are no miracles!!!

MONISTAT AND PRE-NATAL VITAMINS

Okay, yes. Believe it or not, women were going bat crazy behind vaginal cream for hair growth. I guess someone with a yeast infection noticed an incredible bushy growth and there you have it. Clue: If the package does not say it is for hair growth, maybe it should be directed to the area it is needed. The truth is that it works for some, but it is a short term remedy with possible side effects and more hair loss afterwards. However, this will not stop the desperate.

Using a vaginal antifungal cream on your head may cause some hair to possibly break through the scalp where it is thin or balding. Like Emu oil, the vaginal cream wakes up the follicles and allows hair to come through. If the follicles are dead however, by Jesus, it will take a miracle to raise the dead. These are short term remedies and if any hair breaks through, from that point on you are on your own. Neither will grow hair that has already grown.

Nothing has pissed me off more than the great fallacy that prenatal vitamins will grow hair. Prenatal vitamins are for the baby. It is for their brain and spinal cord. If it made hair grow, doctors would have been prescribing it for hair growth for decades, but it does not. At all. "Pre" means before and "natal" means birth. It is as simple as ABC 123, but I have been literally kicked out of a hair group because this knowledge was too much for them.

Does pregnancy effect the hair? Yes, very possibly. When you become pregnant your estrogen level increases and your hair is thrown into part of the resting phase of hair. During that phase, you shed very little hair and your hair may thicken some. Many mothers also know that once the baby is born, for months, you shed that hair until you are back to your normal phase. The thicker hair has nothing to do with prenatal vitamins. The hair is reacting to your body. I went so far as to post an article from the Mayo Clinic, one of the most respected in the world. The article stated that continuing to take prenatal vitamins after giving birth could actually be dangerous to your health, resulting in things like chronic constipation. But, to no avail.

I find it thoroughly amazing how a mind works and the truth gets dropped off like road kill. What people "think" sometimes has absolutely nothing to do with reality. There is a reason that the doctor no longer prescribes them after birth. One who does sees someone before them who is not very bright. They just want to take these women's money. No reputable doctor would do this.

There are some women who do not take prenatal vitamins at all while pregnant. They eat foods that will be beneficial to the baby's brain and spinal column. Their hair still grows at a normal rate. It still thickens and still sheds after birth. Do as you please, but know this: Prenatal vitamins will not make your hair grow! Sad thing is, they truly believe the lies, or as someone else said, "People latch onto a policy or belief and make a conscious decision to not change it. They aren't open to seeing different views."

MY TOP HAIR TIPS FOR NATURAL HAIR GROWTH

From 2012 to 2016. Length checks by flat ironing, but all are natural hair pictures. This took time and care. Not six months, but four years of my normal hair growth.

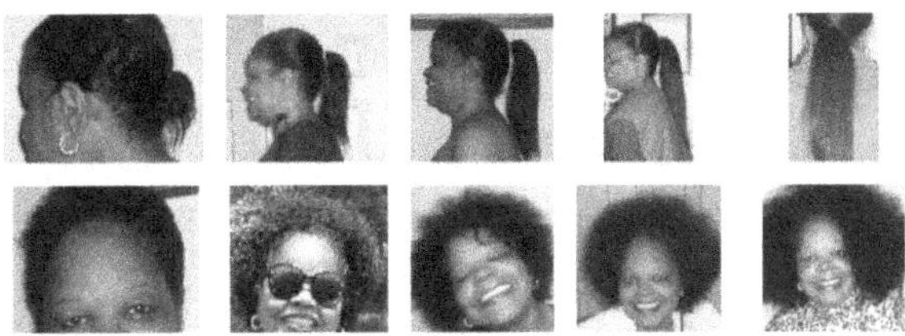

1. Moisturize!

2. Avoid hair knots/fairy knots.

3. Trim dead/split ends.

4. Detangle gently, after moisturizing, from ends upward.

5. Wear a satin or silk cap.

6. Too much manipulation can cause breakage. Try "leave alone" styles.

7. If you wear protective styles, also protect your edges.

8. Stay away from hard gels to prevent circular breakage,

9. Avoid bleaching. Hair becomes brittle and often breaks off.

10. As much as possible, avoid tight braiding, sew-in weaves, and lacefronts as they will lead to traction alopecia, which is sometimes permanent.

I do not feel I should have to tell anyone about weaves, braids and lacefronts and how they can cause permanent damage. We see far too many pictures and videos of hairlines starting at the top of the head and behind the ears. It is hair, not steel. The "I want" of the moment is going to have many in the nursing home one day, all bald. Sometimes we have to think, do "I want" my hair. Be beautiful with natural, relaxed, weaves, or wigs. Be careful with it though. Hair can only take so much, and our hair even less. That is my thing. I am team beautiful, healthy hair.

THE GREAT PRODUCT (I'M LOOKING FOR MY MIRACLE CRAZE)

In truth, I am saddened by what is happening with so many naturals. Some are absolutely clueless and will absolutely not receive knowledge. They look at my hair and you would think they would say, "She must know something." I do, as other professionals also do. I don't know everything, because hair is tricky sometimes. But my success and client success speaks for itself. This does not include all naturals, but far too many.

It is not products that helped me to retain length, but hair care and combing and brushing techniques. Products helped in the health of my hair, but no product made my hair grow. That was taken care of by my mom and dad. Below is a partial list of hair products that cater to natural hair. It is partial because new ones are coming out every day. Giving, sadly, new hope and new disappointment to some. Consider how many years you have been searching, how much money you have spent, and just how much your hair has grown or thrived. Ask yourself, "Am I there yet? Have I reached hair nirvana?"

Every product listed here came from the internet, most from natural hair pages and groups. They are good products depending on your type and texture, but none are miracle workers as wanted by many. The black hair industry is about 700 million dollars a year, not knocking anyone making money, but there are only about

43,000,000 Black Americans. You do the math.

African Pride
African Shea Butter
African Soap
Afro Bella
Afro Sheen
Agadir
Alikay
Alikay Naturals
Aloe Vera
Alter Ego
Ampro
Aphogee
Apple Cider Vinegar
Arganatural Serum
As I Am
Aubrey Organics
Aunt Jackie
Aussie 3 Minute
Miracle
Avanti Silicone Mix
Avlon Kera Care
Baby Don't Be Bald
Be Curly
Beautiful Textures
Moisturizer Butter
Belegenza
Bentonite Clay
Biotin
Black Solutions
Blue Magic
Brazilian Keratin
Bumble and Bumble
Burnt Sugar Pomade
Camille Rose
Cantu
Carol's Daughter
Castor Flaxseed Oil
Chi Silk Infusion
Clay Wash
Coco Conscious
Coconut Vinegar
Come Back Hair
Come Back Hair
Creme
Crème of Nature

Curl Junkie
Curl Keeper
Curls Unleashed
Curly Q's
Darcy's Botanicals
Dark & Lovely
Design Essentials
Devacurl
Diva Chics
Doo Grow
Dove Quench
Absolute
Dr. Bronner Tea Tree
Dr. Miracles
Dudley
E'tae Naturals
Eco Styler
Ed Clarifying
Eden BW
EEOV
Elasta
Elucence
Essentious
EVOO
Fantasia
Fantasia Brazilian
Hair Oil
Fenominaal
Frizz Ease
Fructis
Funky Fro
Giovanni
Glycerin
Going Natural
Gorilla Snot
Gracie's Hair Butter
Greg Juice
Gro Healthy
Groganics
Hair Chemist
Hair Envy
Hair Growth Booster
Hannah Natural
Hawaiin Silky
Hello Curls

Herbal Essence
HG Moisturizer
Hicks
Honey Child
Honeyquat
Hugo Natural
Hydratherma
IC Hair Polish
Indian Healing Clay
Indian Hemp
Infusium 23
It's a 1
It's a Curl (baby)
Jane Carter
JerAki Naturals
JO'M
John Fried Root
Awakening
Kekoa
Kenra
KeraCare Silken Seal
Kinky Curly Knot
Kinky Kudza Knot
Today
Komaya Care
Natureal Curl
Kukoi Oil
Kuku Oil
LeKair Chilesterol
Life Flo Shea Nut Oil
Liquid Castille Soap
Liquid Gold hair
Growth Oil
Lisa Rachel
Loreal
Lottabody Coconut
Milk
Luster Silk Curl
Mane and Tail
Manetabolism
Marshmallow Root
Miss Jessie
Mixed Blessings
Mixed Chicks
Mizani

Moroccanoil
Morrocco Method
Motions
Muhle Organics
Murrays
Naked
Natural Gate
Natural Notts
Naturally Me
Naturalsis 72
Nature Well
Nature's Bounty
Naturelle Grow
Nature's Bounty HSN
Nene's Secret
Not Your Mothers
Nutri Gold Organics
NYC Curls
OBIA
OGX
Ojon
Okay Butters
Olaplex
Olde Jamaica
Optimum Amla
Organic Hair Growth
Booster
Organic Hair
Solutions
Organics Hair Mayo
Organix Coconut
Organix Coconut
Milk
ORS
Ouidad
Palmers
Pantene CoWash
Pattern Pusha Gel
Perfectly Pure
Pink Oil Moisturizer
Queen Beauty
Queen Helene Royal
Curl Shaping Crème
Quemet Biological
Rainforest Chica

Razac
Regrow
Renewing Argan Oil
Renpur
Renpure Originals
Royal Crown
Seda
Shapleys MTG
She
Shea Do
Shea Moisture
Silk Dreams
Simply Organic
Sister Sky Sweet
Grass

Soft & Precious
Soft & Beautiful
Botanicals
Soft & Precious
Softee
Spa Haus
Spectrum
Stay Sof Fro
Strictly Curls
Sulfur8
Super Gro
Super Look
Sweet Potato Souffle
T Gin's Butter Crème
Taliah Waajid Curly

Curl Cream
Tea Tree Tingle
Terressentials
The Mane Choice
The Roots
Trader Joe's Tea
Tree
Tresemme Naturals
Tropic Oil Living
True
Twisted Sista
Twists & Locs
U Be Natural
Ultra Sheen
Moisture Blend

Uncle Funky's
V05
Via Natural
Virgin Hair Fertilizer
Wen
Wetline
Whale Sperm
Wheatgrass Tea
Wild Growth
Xnobe
Yarok
Yes to Carrots
Ylang Ylang
You Be Natural

Is our hair is helpless? This humungous list of hair products seem to indicate that it is. My design is to show that this is going to extremes. It is truly done out of love, tough love, for my people and hopes for better thinking about our hair, about ourselves, and how we treat each other. We should never try and take freedom of choice about anything from black people. We don't need to oppress each other. We have been there in an enormous way. It is not always easy to do natural hair, care for it. But it is worth it if it is your heart's desire, not because someone said you should. However, I am sure that some will use this list of products to make a list of what they need to try, because they still are not getting it.

Take care, gentle care, of your natural hair. IT GROWS!! You simply tear the growth off on the ends. If that one thing could be cemented in our minds, our hair would be better and we would not waste money that could be used in more important arenas.

Finally, I will say this: If you can't or won't wear your root hair the way it truly and naturally is, relaxers never were your problem. If you are natural and filled with venom toward anyone who is not, you are and always have been the problem. Go in. Do I think this book will change things? No. Because far too many will take it as a personal attack. Far too many will be hit dogs that will bare fangs and put up their defense mechanisms. They will go into something that we are chock full of, denial. But it is the truth from my observances. The truth is a hard thing when you have conditioned your brain to lies and this is the ugly truth. The ugly truth is the truth we don't want to face. It is the lies we tell ourselves when we can't face the ugliest truths of all.

www.ingramcontent.com/pod-product-compliance
Lightning Source LLC
Chambersburg PA
CBHW050802240726
48654CB00008B/601